The Four Corners of Disease

The Four Corners
of Disease

Collins C. Conley, Ph.D.

To order additional copies of this book, contact:
Xlibris Corporation
1-888-795-4274
www.Xlibris.com
Orders@Xlibris.com
74484

Contents

Dedicated to my lovely, hardworking, and industrious daughter, Sherry Gordon and her very understanding mother, Eloise Gordon.

Forward

Over the last fifty years there has been a dramatic and rapid decline in the health of the population of the United States. Concomitant with this increase is a skyrocketing increase in the nation's health care costs. In the 1950's it was 5% of the GDP (Gross Domestic Product). From 1960 to 1982 the costs of health care went from $27 billion to $240 billion. Presently, the nation's health care bill is over $2.5 trillion (17 % of the GDP, $7812 per person). The #1 killer in America is cardiovascular disease). There are 1.5 million heart attacks per year resulting in 1 million deaths annually. The #2 killer in America is cancer. 50% of U.S. Citizens will get cancer by age 75 The United States ranks first in sickness among the major industrialized nations. Almost two thirds of the nation is over weight or obese. More than 50% of the nation suffers form chronic illness. The USA ranks 12th in longevity among the major industrialized nations;43rd in infant mortality rate; and 47th in life expectancy. The fundamental causes for this deterioration of the nation's health is (1) the over consumption of refined and processed foods (2)lack of fresh fruits and vegetables in diet (3) over consumption of flesh foods and (4) lack of exercise.

Underscoring the above is the glaring ineffectiveness of traditional western medicine or allopathic medicine as it is commonly called. Its approach is very direct but misguided. Sickness and disease is treated by covering up or masking the symptoms with drugs or employing surgery to remove diseased tissue or organs.

The solution to the nation's health crisis involves a return to a whole foods concept. Many health practitioners over the last 100 years have advocated this approach. Included among these are such men as Dr. Weston Price, Dr. N. W. Walker, Paul C. Bragg, Ph.D., D. C. Jarvis, M.D., Dr. Thomas Powell,

Professor Arnold Ehret and many others. These men advocated diets based upon fresh fruits, vegetables, nuts, seeds, whole grains, beans and possibly very limited quantities of lean meats and/or fresh sea food. Exercise, fresh air, and sunshine are also vital. Food must not be overcooked and must be taken in moderation. Abstention from all drugs is a must—recreational and prescription. All drugs possess dangerous side effects. Annually there are more than 140,000 deaths in the USA from prescription drugs. Another 15-20 thousand deaths occur due to the use of OTC drugs.

The cause of disease can be related to (1) the environment, (2) to one's lifestyle, (3) to one's nutrition and finally (4) to one's genetic makeup. Human beings can exercise a substantial degree of control over the first three causes. Nutrition is the most important of these three. About sixty years ago the key role that nutrition plays in combating disease was uncovered by Dr. Linus Pauling, nobel laureate in chemistry and renown biochemist, Dr. Roger Williams. Dr. Pauling was the first to introduce the concept that disease can originate at the molecular level. That is, disease, can be due to genetic mutations. He further went on to identify possibly the most the critical single nutrient needed by the human body—vitamin C. He went on to quantify the amounts needed by the human body. Dr. Williams was the first to develop the concept called biochemical individuality. This concept recognizes the uniqueness of all individuals at the biochemical level and hence similarly as expressed in the external features. (phenotype). His findings in conjunction with those of Linus Pauling has produced a completely new and vastly improved way of thinking about disease and how to fight it.

The forth, genetics, is largely out of the control of the individual (except possibly for gene expression as it relates to nutrition and the other two factors). Modern science has enabled man to now manipulate the genetic machinery within the cells of the body to cure or ameliorate genetically produced diseases (recombinant DNA technology and gene therapy). This was achieved through the development of the relatively new field of biotechnology. An even more recently developed field called nanotechnology has been combined with biotechnology to produce great promise as a tool to combat human disease at the molecular level. Additionally there exists the considerable promise of stem cell therapy.

This work will focus ostensibly upon the aspects of nutrition as it relates to the generation of health, wellness, vitality and human longevity.

1

Health Status of The United States

The health of the citizens of the USA has steadily declined over the last fifty years. Health care costs are at an all time high. Much of the population is in ill health.

The World Health Organization (WHO), in 2000, ranked the U.S. health care system as the highest in cost, first in responsiveness, 37th in overall performance, and 72nd by overall level of health (among 191 member nations included in the study). A 2008 report by the Commonwealth Fund ranked the United States last in the quality of health care among the 19 compared countries. However, the U.S. is the leader in medical innovation, with three times higher per-capita spending than Europe and producing more new pharmaceuticals, medical devices, and affiliated biotechnology than any other country. The U.S. also has higher survival rates than most other countries for certain conditions, such as some less common cancers, but has a higher infant mortality rate than all other developed countries.

According to the Institute of Medicine of the National Academy of Sciences, the United States is the only wealthy, industrialized nation that does not ensure that all citizens have health insurance coverage. Prescription drug prices in the United States are the highest in the world.

Health Care Expenditures

The United States spends twice as much on health care per capita ($7812) than any other country. For the entire USA this totals to $2.5 Trillion (17.5% of the GDP).

Infant Mortality

The United States ranks 43rd in lowest infant mortality rate, down from 12th in 1960 and 21st in 1990. Singapore has the lowest rate with 2.3 deaths per 1000 live births, while the United States has a rate of 6.3 deaths per 1000 live births. The infant mortality rate is the risk of death during the first year of life, Approximately 30,000 infants die in the United States each year.

Life Expectancy

Life expectancy at birth in the US is an average of 78.14 years, which ranks 47th in highest total life expectancy compared to other countries.

STATUS OF NATIONAL HEALTH

- 20 million with ulcers
- 25 million with asthma
- 120,000 cases of hepatitis
- 24 million cases of diabetes
- 66% of population overweight
- 57 million cases of pre-diabetes
- 600,000 cases of cerebral palsy
- 250,000 cases of multiple sclerosis
- 2.4 million cases of pneumonia yearly
- 46 million arthritics (rheumatoid, gout, lupus, fibromyalgia)
- 200,000 cases of muscular dystrophy
- 1.6 million cancer cases each year
- 25 million cases of heart disease
- 26 million kidney cases in adults
- 27,000 cases of Tuberculosis
- 12 million cases of deafness
- 1.1 million are HIV positive
- 35 million with allergies

Sources: <www.cdc.gov/DataStatistics/;www.Kidney.niddk.nih.
govKudiseases/pubs/Kustats/index.htm>;<www.Seer.cancer.
gov/statfacts/html/all.html>

2

Wholistic Approaches to Health

Wholistic Healing Systems, Diets and Techniques.

There exist many different non-allopathic approaches to combating sickness and disease. They address the nutritional, psychological, physical, mental, emotional and spiritual being of the individual. Some are diets, some are more complex systems or lifestyles; and some are specific healing techniques.

Diets: Vegetarian, fruitarian, raw foods diet, herbal foods diets, fasting, juice diets, mono diets, high fiber diets, low fat diets, high carbohydrate diet

Systems: Macrobiotics, Rosenberg System, Bro. Franco's Bibleway, Ehret System, Jethro Kloss-Back to Eden, Dr. Walker's Health System, and The Adella Davis Approach to Wellness.

Techniques: Acupuncture, reflexology, chiropractic, osteopathy, colon cleansing, water therapy, yoga, massage, iridology, crystal healing, faith healing, homeopathy, biofeedback,. chelation therapy

Some of the more popular and well-known dietary healing systems are:

Professor Arnold Ehret, author of the Mucusless Diet Healing System, was born in 1866 in Germany. He characterizes all diseases as a state of constipation of the human body. A clogging up of the entire pipe system of the body. Disease symptoms merely reflect extraordinary local constipation by accumulated mucus. This mucus is derived from undigested, uneliminated, unnatural and poisonous food substances accumulated in the body over generally a period of many years. The diet consists of all kinds of raw and cooked fruits, starchless vegetables, and cooked or raw mostly green leaf vegetables. This dietary regimen is accompanied by fasting, exercise, fresh air, sunshine, proper bathing, proper sleep and rest.

Jethro Kloss, the author of Back to Eden, was born in 1863 near Manitowoc, Wisconsin. Early in his life he learned that the chemicals and drugs given to sick persons were generally quite dangerous and did not heal. He advocated a return to natural lifestyles. Man's natural diet consists of herbs, fruit, vegetables, nuts and grains. The use of herbs for healing was given special status in his health-generating regime. He was a proponent of fresh air, exercise, physical labor, proper rest, property bathing, pure drinking water, body massage and the use of enemas. As a farmer himself, he advocated proper cultivation and fertilizing of the soil for farms and gardens in order to produce the most nutritious food nature is capable of manufacturing.

N.W. Walker, Ph.D., author of Colon Health and many other books advocates a diet of raw fruits and vegetables and their juices. Dr. Walker found that invariably almost all disease conditions were accompanied by a toxic colon. He agrees that the digestion and assimilation of food comes first, but the lack of elimination of undigested food, waste products, poisons, debris, fermentation and putrefactive products from the colon (and the rest of the body) can result in a complete undermining of ones health. He recommends enemas, proper bathing, pure water and organically grown food.

M.M. Rosenburg, M.D. author of It Is Your Life, advocates a more traditional diet but avoiding excesses of all foods and in particular limiting or eliminating all together refined, processed and chemicalized foods. He would include in a healthy diet, fruits, vegetables, (cooked and raw) meat, fish eggs, poultry, nuts and whole grains. He recommends proper bathing, sleep, exercise, fresh air, sunshine, and a clean home and good posture. Dr. Rosenburg cautions against the taking of drugs and chemical medicines, laxatives, tea, coffee, chocolate, alcohol and tobacco.

Adella Davis, author of Let's Get Well, was one of the country's best-known nutritionists. Throughout her career she worked with many physicians and hospitals helping to restore health to the sick. She planned individual diets for more than 20,000 people suffering from almost every known disease to man. Her approach principally stressed proper nutrition. She included food from all major food groups just as Dr. Rosenburg. She similarly advocated refraining from the use of refined and processed foods. Her opinion is that physicians perform a useful function but they should strongly curtail the use of drugs. She understood their toxic effects and those they induce nutritional deficiencies.

Michie Kushi, author of Natural Healing Through Macrobiotics, asserts that good health is the natural result of maintaining a dynamic balance of ying and yang in our daily eating and life style. Yin and yang, as known in the Orient, are the two basic universal forces, are thought to unlock the secrets of the human body and its relation to the universe. The macrobiotic diet stresses the whole grains (50%) vegetables (30%) and beans/peas and seaweed (15%). The remaining 5% is soup comprised of these three groups. Most of the vegetables are to be cooked and very little fruit or fruit juices are allowed. It does allow for a little fish or roasted seeds or nuts occasionally. It also advocates fresh air, sunshine, exercise, proper bathing and rest.

3

Poor Health in America

The typical American diet consists of approximately 50% concentrated starches and sugars. Grains are processed to produce white flour, white rice, corn grits and oatmeal. These concentrated starches and sugars comprise the breads, cakes, cereals, soft drinks and other sugary beverages, pastas, spaghetti, pastries, sweet fillings and condiments that Americans consume daily. These processed and concentrated sugars are far from the optimum nutrition humans require to promote growth, vitality and optimum health and wellness.

Major Causes of Poor National Health Statistics

- Overconsumption of food
- Overconsumption of meat
- Lack of raw foods and whole foods in diet
- Consumption of processed and refined foods
- Chemical additives, pesticides and preservatives in foodstuffs
- Use of alcohol, tobacco and drugs

It is well known that Eskimos, who exist largely on meats and fat age rapidly with an average life span of 28 years. The Kirgese, a nomadic eastern Russian tribe that lived predominantly on meats, rarely lived past the age of 40. Anthropologists have documented the radiant health, stamina and longevity of several non-meat eating cultures such as the Hunzas of Pakistan, the Ofomi Tribe of Mexico and the Native people of the American Southwest.

It is not uncommon for such tribes to have healthy and active individuals of 110 years of age or more. World Health Statistics consistently show that the nations which consume the most meat have the highest incidence of disease (heart, cancer) and groups of vegetarians in different countries have the lowest incidence of disease. Lastly, the worlds most powerful and greatest stamina possessing and longest-lived animals are all vegetarian. These include the horse, oxen, buffalo, the elephant and others.

Whole Foods

In the thirty years following World War II, the percentage of calories that people derived from stripped down, refined, chemically fabricated and structurally modified food jumped from 10% to 70% of our total diet. When whole foods are modified almost surly their life giving properties are altered in a negative way.

The human body must be supplied with about 46 nutrients from the diet. These nutrients consist of 2 essential fatty acids, 13 vitamins, 17 minerals, 9 amino acids and carbohydrates, water, oxygen, fiber and sunlight. From these nutrients our bodies synthesize about 10,000 different compounds essential to the maintenance of health. Physiological chemists state that there is no blood cell more than 14 days old in the body and that the heart is completely rebuilt every 30 days. The minerals, vitamins and other nutrients necessary for the repair and rebuilding of body cells are found in abundance in fresh, natural whole foods.

NUTRIENT LOSS FROM REFINING OF WHEAT

Nutrient	Per Cent Loss
Cobalt	89
Vitamin E	86
Manganese	86
Magnesium	84
Niacin	81
Riboflavin(B2)	80
Sodium	78
Zinc	78
Potassium	77
Thiamine(B1)	77
Iron	76
Pyridoxine(B6)	72
Phosphorus	71
Calcium	60
Pantothenic Acid (B5)	50
Molybdenum	48
Chromium	40
Selenium	16

Source: Henry A. Schroeder, "Losses of Vitamins and Trace Minerals Resulting from Processing and Preservation of Foods," American Journal of Clinical Nutrition, 1971

A grain kernel is comprised of three layers: the bran, the germ and the endosperm. The bran is the outside layer where most of the fiber exists. The germ is the inside layer where many nutrients and essential fatty acids are found. The endosperm is the starchy middle layer. The high nutrient density associated with grains exists only when these three are intact. The term whole grain refers to the grain before it has been milled into flour. It was not until the late nineteenth century that white bread, biscuits, and cakes made from white flour and sugars became mainstays in the diets of industrialized nations. Dr. Price, a noted dentist, observed the unmistakable consequences of these dietary changes during his travels and documented their corresponding health effects. (Dr Weston. D.D.S. Nutrition and Physical Degeneration. Keats Publishing. 1997.) These changes not only resulted in tooth decay, but problems with fertility, mental health and disease progression.

The Case Against Meat

- **Sick and diseased animals are routinely processed for human consumption.**
- **Animals are highly medicated with drugs such as growth hormones, antibiotics and many others.**
- **Flesh decays very rapidly and poisons the human body if it remains there too long**
- **Meat retains about 13 times more poisons (eg. DDT) than plants.**
- **World statistics show that nations that consume the most meat have the highest incidence of disease while vegetarian nations have the lowest.**
- **Humans have alkaline saliva and much ptyalin to digest grains; meat eaters have acid saliva and no ptyalin.**
- **In man the stomach acid is 20 times weaker than in meat eaters.**

Man is a Plant Eater

Carnivore	Herbivore	Human
Claws	Hands/hoofs	Hands
Sharp teeth	Flat teeth	Flat teeth
Short intestine	Long intestines	Long intestines
Pants to cool body	Sweats to cool body	Sweats to cool body
Manufactures Vitamin C	Diet supplies Vit C	Diet supplies Vit C
No manual dexterity	Hands	Hands
Small brain (limited adaptability of cognitive function	Large brain (able to rationalize)	Large brain (able to reason)

Source: Peter Cox, You Don't Need Meat, Thomas Dunne Books, St. Martin's Press, New York 2002

Selected Drug Nutrient Interactions

Drug	Nutrients Affected
laxatives, mineral oil	calcium, beta carotene, vitamins A, D, K
neomycin (antibiotic)	sodium, potassium, calcium, iron nitrogen, lactose, sucrose, fat, vitamin B12
diuretics, corticosteroids	magnesium, potassium
anti-inflammatory	Iron, Folic acid, vitamin C
oral contraceptives	folic acid, vitamin B6
cholestyramine (lowers cholesterol)	folic acid, iron, vitamins A,D,E,K, B12
salicyates (aspirin)	sodium, potassium, folic acid, vitamin C
alcohol	biotin, cholin, folate, vitamins A,B1,B3,B12
steroids (prednisone)	vitamins B6,C,D
Tetracycline (antibiotic)	calcium, potassium, magnesium, iron, biotin, inositol, vitamins B1,B2,B3,B6,B12

Sources: Robert H. Garrison, Jr. ;M.A.R. Ph., Elizabeth Summer, M.A. The Nutrition Desk Reference 1985; J.E. Wiliams, O. M.D. Prolonging Health, Hampton Roads Publishing Co, Inc., 2003

4

Biochemical Individuality and the Genetic Basis for Disease

The term "biochemical individuality" was first popularized by Roger Williams. (see reference in table below) Its coinage and usage grew out of a most intriguing conjecture by two time Nobel Laureate in chemistry and peace Linus Pauling in his landmark article on the mechanism of the production of sickle cell anemia published in 1949. He proposed the term "molecular medicine". It proposed a new origin of disease based on the recognition that specific mutations of the genes can create an altered "molecular environment" and hence an altered physiological function producing a disease state in the human body. Pauling had been working on the general problem of the relation of physiological activity to molecular structure of substances present in the human body. Since physiological activity is controlled by the structure, altered physiology then must originate and be controlled by genes. This was a bold step taken by Linus Pauling. but such is necessary for advances in science. His conjecture has since been proven true.

Roger Williams, a biochemist, took note of Pauling's work. His pioneering work in biochemistry, nutrition science and molecular biology have played a major role in our understanding the molecular origin of disease. This understanding is exemplified in the concept of biochemical individuality. Residing at the center of this concept is the all controlling life machinery itself—the human gene. Over the last thirty years as the molecular biology of the gene has become well understood it has become clear that almost certainly almost all diseases are rooted in the vast variability of our genes.

Scientists have made the connection between the gene and nutritional requirements, environment and life styles. These three interaction greatly affect our overall health. They modulate/control to a certain degree the transformation of one's genotypes into phenotypes (outward physical characteristics and capabilities).

Dr. Williams coined the term "genotrophic disease" to describe diseases resulting from genetically based nutrition or metabolic needs that are not being met. Because of the vast variability of genes he put forth the proposition that we are all biochemical unique and should be recognized by the medical profession as such when treating disease. He along with many others have asserted that the RDA's, which address normal nutritional needs have little or no relevancy to the concept of optimum nutrition for individual needs or to the treatment of disease states.

Ranges for Selected Human Paramaters

Parameter	Range (high/low)	Ratio
Size of Stomach	—	8
Size of Liver	—	4
Heart rates in men	105/45	2.33
Total leucocyte count in healthy adult	14800/3500	4.23
Enzyme production	—	50
Vitamin A(carotene) in human blood	300/20	15
Pumping capacity of heart	10.81/3.16	3.42
Water composition of female	70.2%/45.6%	1.54
Inorganic Flourine in blood plasma	45/10	4.5
Inorganic Zinc in blood plasma	613/0	—
Glycogen in blood	16.2/1.2	13.5
Amino acid Glycine in blood	5.4/.8	6.75
Endocrine gland hormone levels	—	10

Source: Compiled from Roger Williams Ph.D., Biochemical Individuality, Keats Publishing, New Canaan, Conneticut, 1998

Vitamin C Requirements in Humans

Disease or Condition	Amount of Vitamin (milligrams per day)
Scruvy prevention	5-15
RDA (adult male)	90
Optimum value for good health[a] for most humans	1000-3000
Optimum Value for good health[b] for most humans	2500+
Optimum value for good health[c] for most humans according to Linus Pauling	2000-4000
Range of human needs based on biochemical individuality according to Linus Pauling	250-10,000
Amounts used in orthomolecular medicine (therapeutic level)	30,000-40,000 and even 1000,000

[a]Dr. Emanuel Cheraskin, Dr. W. Marshall Ringsdorf Jr., Dr. Emily L. Sisley. Harpers and Row Publishers, New York, 1983.

[b]Steve Hickey Ph.D., Hilliary Roberts Ph.D., Pauling Vindicated; Researchers Claim RDA for Vitamin C is Flawed. <http:www2. prnewswire.com/cgi—bin/stories.pl?ACCT=109&STORY=/www/ story/07-06 . . . 9/29/2009

[c]Linus Pauling, Vitamin C the Common Cold and the Flu, W.H. freeman and Company,1976.

Steve Hickey and Hilliary Roberts, both pharmacology professors challenge the RDAs set by the Institute of Medicine and the National Institutes of Health, They assert that the values of 90 mg and 75 mg for men and women respectively are based on flawed science and are much too low. The basis for the claim is the fact that the half life of vitamin C in the human body is thirty minutes. Given this short half life, tests must be conducted immediately after a dosage of the vitamin is given, not twelve hours later as has been done. Hickey and Roberts findings suggest that a minimum of 2500mg of vitamin C be taken in divided doses throughout the day in order to establish proper levels of the vitamin in the blood plasma. Given the short half life of thirty minutes it should be taken daily in divided doses around the clock for optimum health and wellness. (given that B vitamins are not stored in the body this might apply to them also) This can be accomplished by the use of time released supplements. Their work validates the long held claims of Linus Pauling that high doses of several grams and more are needed for optimal health and well being. It also supports the clinical findings of Dr. Fredrick Klenner that vitamin C is highly effective against many viral and bacterial infections.

5

Strategies for Healing Your Body

1. Caloric Restriction

Clive M. McCay, a nutritional scientist at Cornell University in the 1930's sought to determine if calorie restriction could extend lifespan. He successfully demonstrated this with rodents. He fed a group of rats 40% less calories and found that it extended lifespan 40-50%. This increase in life span was accompanied with an onset of sterility. The diet also delayed the onset of diseases related to aging such as cancer, heart disease and brain diseases.

Another well document study of calorie restriction was carried out on Japanese in Okinawa. Children and adults consumed 20-30% fewer calories than the national average. Death rates from cancer, stroke and heart disease were lower by about 60%. The number of centenarians on the island was forty times greater than that of northeast Japan where calorie intake was normal.

Since the early work of McCay at Cornell many other researchers have carried out studies that confirm his results.

About twenty five years ago researcher at UC Irvine, UCSF and MIT discovered that specific sets of genes in lab animals kept cells from wearing out or being overwhelmed by free radicals,. Such genes are capable of controlling or altering the rate of aging. The researchers further discovered that this gene(s) could be activated by caloric restriction and other stresses. (see Joseph Maroon M.D., The Longevity Factor, Atria Books, New, York NY, 2009)

It was discovered that certaind chemical substances found in common foods could mimic caloric restriction and activate these longevity genes. Resveratrol, a substance found in grapes, which belongs to a class of chemical compounds called polyphenols, could activate these longevity genes. Caloric restriction is not involved at all. Resveratrol is the most potent polyphenol found to date.

By combining caloric restriction with a diet of polyphenol containing plants one would expect the longevity genes to activated to a greater extent with possibly with a synergistic effect present.

Year Life	Expectance (yrs)	Attributed To
1796	25	poor sanitation, diets
1896	48	poor sanitation, diets
2009 (actual)	80	poor diets, alcohol, cigarettes, drugs, toxins in food and environment
2009[a] (predicted)	100-120	caloric restriction, diet, life style, supplements
Bible (Genesis 6:3) and Hayflick limit	120	God; calculation by Dr. Leonard Hayflick
2029[b]	120-150	biotechnology, stem cells, nanotechnology. hormone replacement therapy

[a]This author by application of caloric reduction to humans coupled with latest knowledge of nutrition and nutritional supplement.

[b]Dr. Ronald Klatz, Dr. Robert Goldman, Basic Health Publications, Inc., 2003.

2. Enzymes

Enzymes are killed or denatured at sustained temperatures above 118 F. When food deprived of its natural enzymes is consumed by humans the human body must produce more of its own endogenous enzymes to digest the food. Overworking of the body in this manner leads to decreased production of the body's own metabolic enzymes. All glands and major organs suffer. The brain shrinks, the pancreas swells and other organs enter a survival mode characterized by certain abnormalities.

To optimize one's health and life span, the diet should include a generous proportion of raw food. The proportion will vary depending upon the individual, their lifestyle, their environment and their genetic makeup. Cooked food should be limited to 15 to 30 per cent of one's diet. As the amount of food in the diet is reduced then the proportion of cooked food can be more safely increased.

3. Cooked Versus Raw Food

Bonding between glucose molecules and proteins leads to the buildup of glucose molecules on protein surfaces. Dubbed Advanced Glycosylation Endproducts (*AGEs*), these glucose-protein complexes are also thought to lead to the formation of protein crosslinks as multiple proteins become associated with the AGE complex. These crosslinks are thought to be a major marker and possible impetus in aging in general An often cited example of crosslinking being the wrinkling of the skin. This process of glucose molecules and proteins bonding together occurs naturally within the human body. Many proteins must undergo this translation process in order that they may become fully physiologically active in the body. Vitamin C and selenium help protect against this process.

A potentially cancer-causing agent used to manufacture certain chemicals, plastics, and dyes has now been found to be a natural by-product of cooking certain foods. The FDA is taking a closer look at this white, odorless chemical, acrylamide, to determine how much of it occurs in foods and whether it could pose a health risk to consumers. (<http://www.acrylamide.org>)

Researchers in Sweden discovered that cooking at high temperatures could create acrylamide in many types of foods, particularly starchy foods such as french fries, potato chips, bread, rice, and processed cereals. Scientists know that acrylamide causes cancer in laboratory rats. They also know contact with large quantities of acrylamide can cause nerve damage in humans. Acrylamide was not found in uncooked or boiled food. Studies indicate that it forms during high temperature (greater than 250 F) cooking processes, such as frying and baking, and that levels of acrylamide increase with heating time. Based on high-dose experiments in animals, acrylamide is classified as a potential human carcinogen, as well as a genotoxicant, a substance that can mutate and damage genetic material.

The World Health Organization, the U.S. Food and Drug Administration (FDA) and California's Office of Environmental Health Hazard Assessment (OEHHA) have studied the issue. OEHHA has gathered data and published a report which includes estimates of acrylamide levels for 40 foods. Given that assessment, it is estimated that consumers of french fries receive up to 125 times the amount of acrylamide that requires a warning under current regulations, while consumers of potato chips receive as much as 75 times the level requiring a warning. The report is available online at <www.oehha. ca.gov/prop65/acrylamideqa.html>.

Raw Versus Cooked Food

	Cooked	Raw
Enzymes (beneficial)	**destroyed near 118 F**	present
Vitamins (beneficial)	**many destroyed**	present
Minerals (beneficial)	**possibly denatured by heat**	present
Fiber (beneficial)	**heat breaks down fiber**	present
Polyphenols (beneficial)	**heat destroys**	present
Acrylamide (toxic)	present	none
AGEs (toxic)	present	none

4. Raw Fruit and Vegetable Juices

Nourishment for the body is derived from the food that we consume. This nourishment goes to build and revitalize the trillions upon trillions of individual cells that comprise the physical structure, This structure is not permanent. It is continuously being broken down (catabolism) by the wear and tear of action and simultaneously built up (anabolism) by the process of repair. No cell in the human body is more than seven years old; no blood cell is more than fourteen days old; and a new heart is built every thirty days, Cells from the small intestine walls are replaced every forty eight hours. The complete set of nutrients required to construct and maintain the human body can be found only in raw foods.

The cooking of foods will destroy a number of food factors. (e,g. vitamins, enzymes, cysteine). In addition to this, cooked food will possess certain harmful properties. Enzymes are harmed when food is cooked. They are completely destroyed above 118 degrees Fahrenheit. This is most serious as enzymes are the fundamental driving force behind all life processes. They make possible all work done at the cellular level within the human body They act as catalyst for the many biochemical reactions that occur within the human body. These God-given enzymes are locked within the plant fibers,

Thorough mastication is required for their release for utilization by the body. This applies equally well to vitamins, minerals and other nutrients. However, there is one drawback even beyond mastication The tough cellulose wall of the plant fiber can not be digested by the human digestive system. This is not all bad as these fibers can physically clean debris and waste matter from the human colon. Cooked food leaves a glue-like coating on the colon walls.

To obtain immediate nutrition from plants without consumption of the fibers, the plants must be taken in the form of virgin, raw juices. These raw juices enter the blood stream in ten to fifteen minutes. The whole raw vegetables would require three to five hours of processing These raw juices are extremely perishable and should be consumed within minutes of preparation.

5. Vitamin C and the Anti-stress Factors

A Historical Perspective

Vitamin C has been found to be possibly the single most important vitamin needed by the human body. (other than air and water) Of course anytime a vitamin C deficiency is present there are many deficiencies with respect to other nutrients. This deficiency surfaced as a result of long sea going voyages in the 18th century during which no fresh fruits or vegetables were among the staples carried along. The crews subsisted ostensibly on salt pork, salt beef and biscuits,

After 2-3 months at sea the crew began to experience ulcerated gums follows by falling out of ones teeth, physical weakness, muscle pain, diarrhea, pulmonary and kidney troubles followed by eventual death. On long voyages sometimes as much as two thirds of the crew would perish from scurvy. Case in point is that of Vasco da Gamma, who was first to discover that by sailing around the southern tip of Africa, that one could reach India. One hundred of his crew of one hundred sixty died of scurvy on the voyage.

Scurvy has also plagued other groups in addition sailors on long voyages. It has broken out amongst soldiers on campaigns, within communities when food is scarce, in cities under siege and in prisons.

The cause of scurvy was found in 1747 by a Scottish physician working in the service of the British navy named James Lind M.D. He carried out a now famous experiment with twelve patients ill with scurvy. He placed them all on the same diet except for one item, To each of two patients he gave two oranges and one lemon per day; to two others, cider; to the others, dilute sulfuric acid or vinegar; or sea water or a mixture of drugs. At the end of six days the two that had received the oranges an lemon were well, but the other ten were still ill. He carried out further studies and published his findings in a book in 1753 entitled a Treatise on Scurvy. However, it took until 1795 for the British command to order rations of citrus to all sailors in the British navy When this occurred all scurvy disappeared from the British navy

This finding by Lind raised the question as to whether or not there are poisons in certain foods or are their certain protective substances in certain foods. The answer was provided in 1911 by Casmir Funk a Swedish biochemist. He published his theory of "vitamins" which explained that their exist natural substances found in foods that protect against diseases such as beriberi, scurvy, pellagra and rickets. Scientists began to search for the anti-scorbutic vitamin—vitamin C.

It was finally isolated in 1928 by a scientist Albert Szent-Gyorgyi. The chemical formula for vitamin C is $C_6H_8O_6$. Since only a few particular foods containing vitamin C do prevent scurvy, it can be inferred that vitamin C works in conjunction with other undiscovered food factors or nutrients present only in these few select foods. The full list of foods that prevent a vitamin C deficiency is as follows:

Foods Preventing a Vitamin C Deficiency

Citrus

Potatoes

Grape Juice

Green Leaves

Onions

Vitamin C functions within the body to

- Enhance the absorption of iron (intravenous does not work most foods do not work)
- Neutralizes chlorine in drinking water (chlorine cripples red blood cells)
- Enhances immunity
- Protects the heart
- Is a natural anesthetic
- Lowers fat and cholesterol levels
- Helps detoxify heavy metals (lead, cadmium, nickel, mercury, arsenic, fluorides, aluminum) and poisons (carbon monoxide, alcohol, benzene, chloroform. carbon tetrachloride, cyanides, nicotine, ozone) and ionizing radiation.
- Reduces insulin requirements for diabetics
- Helps fight cancer
- Slows aging

Vitamin C is destroyed within the body by

- aspirin
- cigarettes
- OTC drugs
- sleeping pills
- contraceptives
- carbonated beverages
- many prescription drugs
- caffeine
- alcohol

Vitamin C Production in Selected Mammals

Animal	Milligrams/Kg Body Weight/per Day	Man's Equivalent per Day in milligrams
Mouse	275	19,250
Rabbit	226	15,820
Goat	190	13,300
Rat	150	10,500
Dog	40	2800
Cat	40	2800

Source: "Why We Need to Supplement Our Vitamin C Intake."<www.Cforyourself.com/ Overview/Primer/ what_C_Does/why_take_c.l>()

Notice that dogs and cats are low producers (relatively) and that they are more susceptible to vitamin C deficiency related problems. However, man, apes, fruit bats, guinea pigs and some species of fish do not make vitamin C. The column headed man's equivalent shows how much a 150 pound person would produce at the rate of that animal. As you can see it is totally reasonable that at least three grams per day might be required by man for good health It is also reasonable due to biochemical individuality that some segment of the population might require as much as ten to even twenty grams per day to remain well or attain optimal health.

Vitamin C as a Therapeutic Agent

Fredrick R. Klenner M.D. conducted pioneering studies that confirmed the ability of vitamin C to cure many viral and bacterial infections and poisons He concludes that vitamin C is the single most important nutrient for achieving and maintaining optimal health.

Klenner Type Treatments for Selected Viral Diseases

Disease	Effectiveness	Dosage
Measles	Curable, Preventable	1000 mg very 2 hrs by mouth around the clock for 4 days
Mumps	Curable, Preventable	25,000 mg total over 60 hrs intravenously
Pneumonia	Curable, Preventable	1000 mg every 6 to 12 hrs intravenously
Chicken Pox and Herpes	Curable, Preventable	2000 to 3000 mg intravenously every 12 hrs and1000 mg orally every 2 hrs ; total of 6 injections; cured in 72 hrs
Encephalitis	Curable, Preventable	6000 mg intravenously every 6 hrs; a 10,000 mg dose orally and recovery complete in 24 hrs
Hepatitis	Curable, Preventable	120,000 mg per day orally over 4 days
Polio	Curable, Preventable	6,000 to 20,000 mg per day intravenously;50,000 to 80,000 mg orally per day

Source: Compiled from Thomas E. Levy M.D., J.D., Vitamin C, Infectious Disease and \ Toxins, Philadelphia, PA, Exlibris Corp. 2002.

Adella Davis, the first of the new age health enthusiast, utilized the healing qualities of food factors that she called the antistress factors. The antistress factors are vitamin-like substances that are yet unidentified by modern science. They provide a high level of protection from many but not all forms of stress. When rats are given such toxic substances as strychnine, sulfanilamide, cortisone, promine or even aspirin they all cause much harm that cannot be arrested by any known vitamin, mineral or other nutrient. When foods supplying the antistress factors are given the rats are completely protected. See Adella Davis, Let's Get Well, Harcourt Brace Janovich, Inc., 1965 and references therein.

The antistress factors are found in several foods listed below.

Anti-Stress Foods

Liver

Wheat Germ

Yeast

Soy Flour

Kidneys

Green Leaves

6.   Constipation and Colon Health

Constipation, in general, relates to the elimination of toxins (endogenous as well as exogenous), dead or decaying body cells or tissues and foreign microbes and other matter from the human body. Within the body are seven channels of elimination,. These are the bowels, kidneys, lungs, skin, blood, liver, and lymphatic system. All of these may become clogged up and hence what we might call constipated. The arterial system as well as the entire body can become constipated. When constipated the body organs including the organs of elimination will not properly carry out their physiological functions. Disease is ostensibly a state in which the entire human body is clogged up or constipated.

This section will focus on constipation of the colon or bowels. It focuses on the lack of proper elimination of fecal matter from the colon. There are several types of constipation. (see Robert Gray, The Colon Health Handbook, Emerald Publishing 1986)

Types of Constipation

1. Constipation, as thought of by the average lay person is the lack of sufficient bowel movements.
2. One is said to be constipated also when the bowels do move but the feces are hard or compacted. Hard and compacted stools signify unnatural and possibly diseased conditions within the body.
3. Constipation also refers to the condition within the body whereby bowel movements do occur but hard compacted fecal matter coats the inner walls of the colon. The origin of this compacted material will be explained below.
4. Diarrhea, according to Robert Gray can be considered a form of constipation.

There are a number of contributory causes to constipation within the human body. One of the primary causes is due to mucoid deposited within the colon by mucoid forming foods. Mucoid or mucus as it is also sometimes called is also secreted by certain glands within the body. This mucoid matter is secreted in an effort to encapsulate invading toxins, bacteria, viruses, bacteria or dust particles. Mucoidal substances are slimly and sticky by nature. The presence of mocoidal matter in a human stool will slow the passage of the feces through the colon and out of the body as compared to a mucoidless stool. These mucoidal substances deposit a layer of slimy material onto the inner walls of the colon. This material can become hardened over time. Once this happens it can prevent the transfer of nutrients across the colon wall. It also prevents the passage of toxins from the body into the colon for elimination from the body. This situation leads to long transit times for the food. Typically transit times for people in the USA range from three to six days. On a healthy and low mucoidal diet this should be one day. These long transit times that typically plague Americans lead to putrefaction and autointoxication. Putrefaction is indicated by the presence of rotting, decaying, poison ladened, microbe infested, foul smelling feces. This putrid material can then be absorbed into the body resulting in what is termed autointoxication. Foods that are mucoidless or possess very low mucoid forming potential include almost all fruits, vegetables, sprouts, nuts and seeds, and herbs. Most grains and beans will be mucoid forming. Flesh foods such as meat, fish, fowl and eggs are highly mucoid forming. Dairy products such as milk, butter, cheese, cottage cheese, yogurt, cream and others are the most mucoid forming foods of all.

Combating Constipation

1. Adopt a mucoidless forming diet (fruits, vegetables, nuts, seeds, herbs)
2. Consume lots of fluids (fruit juices, vegetable juices, herbal teas/juices and water)
3. Increase the vitamin C intake (two to four grams is the range for optimal health but more may be required)
4. Reduce the caloric intake. Only one or two meals a day. Begin by eating one meal one day out of each week. And over time strive to increase this to two and then to three and so on. You will reach a limit based upon your will power, the strength and adequately of your diet and the principle of biochemical individuality.

Indicators of Proper Colon Functioning

1. No putrefaction
   (no odorous or foul smelling elimination)
   (apples are excellent at combating putrefaction)
   (minimize flesh foods and dairy and drinking with meals)
   (generous amounts of raw foods)
2. Minimize fermentation
   (minimize consumption of refined and processed carbohydrates.)
   (consume more foods low in carbohydrates)
   (Honey can help stop fermentation. Practically all honeys contain sugar-tolerant yeast. These sugar-tolerant yeast remain largely inactive at temperatures of 50 F or less or if the moisture content of the honey is less than about 18 per cent. Granulated honeys are less resistant to fermentation.)
3. Transit time of one day
   (the following possess laxative properties: vitamin C supplements, spinach, grape juice, honey, a mixture of prune juice/apple sauce/bran, a warm glass of sauerkraut juice followed by a warm glass of grapefruit juice)
4. Eliminations approximately mirror the number of meals
   (if the number of eliminations is less then the number of meals each day then reduce the number of meals while increasing fluids.)
5. Gastrocolic Reflex Action
   (taking of a meal produces a bowel movement usually within ten to fifteen minutes)
   (a bowel movement should occur upon rising in the morning)

7. Nutritional Supplements

The human body requires certain nutrients that it must rely upon from the diet. Among the most important of these are vitamins A, C, E (antioxidants), vitamin D (bone and cellular health) and vitamin B12 (antiaging, DNA synthesis, nerve health).

Nutrient	RDA (daily)	Max Safe Level
Vitamin A	3000 IU (men) 2000 IU (women)	25,000 IU (short term) 10,000 IU (long term), pregnant or diseased consult doctor
Vitamin C	90 mg for men 75 mg for women women women	Virtually non toxic
Vitamin D	*men and women* 200 IU infant to 50 yrs 400 IU 51 to 70 yrs 600 IU over 70 yrs	1000 IU advisable; 800 IU pregnant or breast feeding
Vitamin D[a]	1000 IU (recommended)	All over age 1
Vitamin E	15 IU men 12 IU women	800 IU long and short term
Vitamin B12	2.4 mcg men and women 2.6 mcg pregnant 2.8 mcg lactating	3000 mcg generally accepted; virtually nontoxic

[a]Michael F. Holick, Ph. M.D., Mark Jenkins, The UV Advantage, iBooks, Inc. 2003

Of these above nutrients vitamins C and D are considered to be the two most important to good health. Vitamin C is the most important with vitamin D being second. Vitamin D will be discussed below as vitamin C has been addressed already in this work.

Vitamin D sufficiency, along with diet and exercise, has emerged as one of the most important preventive factors in human health. Hundreds of studies now link vitamin D deficiency with significantly higher rates of many forms of cancer, as well as heart disease, osteoporosis, multiple sclerosis and many other conditions and diseases. (see reference a in above table)

Vitamin D is essential for promoting calcium absorption in the gut and maintaining adequate serum calcium and phosphate concentrations to enable normal mineralization of bone and prevent hypocalcemic tetany. It is also needed for bone growth and bone remodeling by osteoblasts and osteoclasts. Without sufficient vitamin D, bones can become thin, brittle, or misshapen. Vitamin D sufficiency prevents rickets in children and osteomalacia in adults. Together with calcium, vitamin D also helps protect older adults from osteoporosis.

Vitamin D has other roles in human health, including modulation of neuromuscular and immune function and reduction of inflammation. Many genes encoding proteins that regulate cell proliferation, differentiation, and apoptosis are modulated in part by vitamin D.

Vitamin D is a fat-soluble vitamin that is naturally present in very few foods, added to others, and available as a dietary supplement. It is also produced endogenously when ultraviolet rays from sunlight strike the skin and trigger vitamin D synthesis. Vitamin D obtained from sun exposure, food, and supplements is biologically inert and must undergo two hydroxylations in the body for activation. The first occurs in the liver and converts vitamin D to 25-hydroxyvitamin D [25(OH)D], also known as calcidiol. The second occurs primarily in the kidney and forms the physiologically active 1,25-dihydroxyvitamin D [1,25(OH)$_2$D], also known as calcitriol. Scientific research has found that all cells and tissues in your body have vitamin D receptors that can convert these precursors directly into the active form of vitamin D. further it has been found that every cell and tissue needs vitamin D for its well-being.

Research suggests that up to 85% of people could be deficient in vitamin D without knowing it . . . leaving them with less-than-optimal health. In fact, some scientists call for urgent action.

Vitamin D is responsible for the regulation of over 2,000 genes in your body. Vitamin D engages in very complex metabolic processes within your body. Scientists believe that vitamin D serves a wide range of fundamental biological functions relating to many aspects of your health.

Exposure to vitamin-D-producing UVB light can vary greatly depending upon many factors, including time of day and year; and the latitude, altitude, and prevailing weather conditions of where we live. Latitude is especially important. Season, geographic latitude, time of day, cloud cover, smog, skin melanin content, and sunscreen are among the factors that affect UV radiation exposure and vitamin D synthesis. The UV energy above 37 degrees north latitude (a line between San Francisco, CA and Richmond, VA) is insufficient for cutaneous vitamin D synthesis from November through February ; in far northern latitudes, this reduced intensity lasts for up to 6 months. In the United States, latitudes below 34 degrees north (a line between Los Angeles, CA and Columbia, SC) allow for cutaneous production of vitamin D throughout the year.

For people with a low melanin content 10 to 15 minutes daily on their hands, face and arms Is sufficient to make enough vitamin D provided exposure is at a latitude at or below 34 degrees. As the latitude increases of course the exposure time must correspondingly increase. Similarly for dark skinned persons of African descent 30 minutes to 3 hours may be required.

According to Dr. Holick the vitamin D produced by the sun contains a range of different photoproducts. Vitamin D from food or supplements would not necessarily be totally equivalent and hence they would not yield the same health benefits. Hence, one should always obtain as much of their daily supply of vitamin D from the sunshine.

Natural sources of vitamin D include:cod liver oil, herring,catfish, salmon, mackerel,sardines, tuna, eel, egg, beef liver.

The practical reality is that on average, the U.S. diet provides 100 IU/day. One problem is that much of the fortified milk is not fortified to the required amount and many people do not drink milk.

Serum concentration of 25(OH)D is the best indicator of vitamin D status. It reflects vitamin D produced cutaneously and that obtained from food and supplements and has a fairly long circulating half-life of at least 15 days. Because of this relatively long half life it is possible for the vitamin D to build up to toxic levels in the body and result in death. (this was not the case with vitamin c as it has a short half life of only thirty minutes) However, it is not possible to produce toxic levels of vitamin D in the body from that produced by the sunshine, only. Vitamin D produce this way self destructs after it has been utilized by the cells and hence no amount of sun exposure alone can produce vitamin D toxicity.

Super Foods

In addition to the above supplements of vitamins A,C, D,E and B12 the author uses and recommends such super foods as honey, lemons, grape juice, apple cider vinegar, kelp, blackstrap molasses, liver, onions and garlic. The best sources for B vitamins are such high potency foods as wheat germ, liver (very high in B12), rice polishings, and brewers yeast. Wheat germ, whole grains, and nuts and seeds are good sources of vitamin E. The only good source of vitamin A is fish liver oils. The author recommends supplementation of the essential fatty acids by using olive oil and canola oil.

8. Exercise, Fresh Air and Sunshine

Exercise

- — increases muscle mass
- — increase oxygenation of the cells
- — promote the elimination of toxins through sweating
- — move waste products through the lymphatic vessels help return used blood through the veins (which have no
- — muscles or pump of their own)
- — stimulate immune function
- — improve bowel function
- — strengthen bones

Sunlight

- • strengths the blood
- • improves the mood
- • makes the bones stronger

- helps prevent internal cancers
- helps in healing skin diseases such as psoriasis
- strengthens the immune system
- improves the heart function
- regulates blood sugar
- prevents tooth decay

Daylight is essential for good health because of its beneficial affect on hormone balance. Your brain requires a certain amount of natural light each and every day. The natural light that hits your retina (light gathering area inside the eye) is transmitted to an area of your brain called the pineal body. The pineal is the brain center for the production of the hormone melatonin. Melatonin regulates daily body rhythms, most notably the day/night cycle (circadian rhythms). Normal melatonin levels are important for natural sleep cycles and proper immune system function

Benefits of oxygen

- kills bacteria and viruses
- improves functioning of cilia in lungs
- lowers body temperature
- improves sense of well being
- tranquilizing relaxing

Fresh air is chemically different than the re-circulated indoor air that most people breathe. High quality fresh air is actually electrified. The oxygen molecule is negatively charged.

9. A Biblical Based Diet

In the beginning man's diet consisted of fruits only.

Genesis 1:29
And God said, Behold, I have given you every herb yielding seed, which is upon the face of all the earth, and every tree, in which is the fruit of a tree yielding seed; to you it shall be for food.

Later, God added vegetables to man' diet.

Genesis 1:30
And to every beast of the earth, and to every fowl of the air, and to every thing that creepeth upon the earth, wherein there is life, I have given every green herb for meat: and it was so.

After the flood the earth's soil and climate was dramatically changed. In many places on earth it would not be possible to obtain enough food from plant sources during all times of the year. It was at this time that God gave man permission to each animal flesh. Yet even in this God gave instruction that the blood must be drained from the carcass before eating it.

Genesis 9:3
Every moving thing that liveth shall be meat for you; even as the green herb have I given you all things.

Genesis 9:4
But flesh with the life thereof, which is the blood thereof, shall ye not eat.

The bible diet is largely influenced by Jewish dietary law, the rules for determining clean and unclean foods are derived from certain passages from the bible. Clean foods are those which in their natural state do not harm the human body and which man can use for his nourishment. Unclean foods are those which are unhealthy to consume and are poisonous to the body. The primary passages regarding man' s proper diet are Leviticus 11 and Deuteronomy 14. Others include Genesis, Proverbs, Luke, Paul, Exodus, Peter, Judges, Isaiah, Corinthians, Habakkuk, and Daniel. Physical, mental and spiritual health are all highly dependent upon man consuming a correct and proper diet. Animals are divided into the following categories:

- Mammals
- Birds
- Reptiles
- Water animals
- Insects

Clean mammals are:

1) cloven-footed
2) parteth the hoof
3) chew the cud

Unclean	swine, hare, camel, musrat, boar, horse, donkey, squirrel, rabbit, raccoon, bear, opossum mule, beaver, badger porcupine
Clean	cattle, deer, goat, ox, bison, elk sheep, antelope, elk, moose, caribou, gazelle

Forbidden birds include: carnivores, scavengers, crows, buzzards, bats, owls, eagles, sea gulls, hawks, herons, falcons, ostriches, suffrage, cuckow, ospray, herons, storks, ravens, pelicans, vultures and no fowls on all fours creeping.

Birds safe to ear include: chicken, duck, pigeon, swan, goose, quail, turkey, partridge, pheasant, grouse, sparrow, guinea fowl, prairie chicken, dove

All reptiles are banned. This means all snakes and snake-like creatures that go upon the belly or on all fours or have many legs: frog, toad, crocodile, lizard, snake, turtle, salamander, newt, snail.

Fish are clean if they have fins and scales.

Unclean: crabs, lobsters, shrimp, oysters, catfish, eel, seal, walrus, shark, swordfish, squid, mussel, whale, shark, scallop, marlin, octopus, dolphin, otter, porpoise, crayfish, clams.

Clean : flounder, striped bass, red snapper, halibut, haddock, buffalo, trout, tilapia, mackerel, salmon, herring carp, sardine, whiting, cod

Very few insects are clean and may be eaten by man. These include grasshoppers, beetles, and locust.

The Human Body is the Temple of God

1 CORINTHIANS 10:31
Whether therefore ye eat, or drink, or whatsoever ye do, do all to the glory of God.

1 CORINTHIANS 3:16, 17
Know ye not that ye are the temple of God, and that the Spirit of God dwelleth in you? If any man defile the temple of God, him shall God destroy; for the temple of God is holy, which temple ye are.

1 CORINTHIANS 6:19, 20
What? know ye not that your body is the temple of the Holy Ghost which is in you, which ye have of God, and ye are not your own? For ye are bought with a price: therefore glorify God in your body, and in your spirit, which are God's.

Appendix

The Essential Nutrients for the Human Body

Essential Fatty Acids: lenoleic, lenolenic

Amino Acids: histidine, leucine, lysine, isobutene, threonine, tryptophan methionine, valine, Phenylalanine

Vitamins: A (retinol), B1(thiamine), B2(riboflavin), B3(niacin), B5(pantithetic acid), B6(pyridoxine), B12(cyanocobalamine), folic acid, biotin, C, D, E, K.

Minerals: calcium, magnesium, phosphorus, potassium, sodium, sulfur, iron, zinc, copper, manganese, chromium, selenium, cobalt, flourine, silicon, iodine, molybdenum.

Others: carbohydrates, fats, light, oxygen, water, exercise

Dr. Collins C. Conley is a physical chemist. He received his doctorate form Cornell University in the area of molecular spectroscopy. His undergraduate studies were conducted at Clark Atlanta University (formerly Clark College) located in Atlanta, GA. Postdoctoral studies in laser spectroscopy were carried out at Howard University in Washington, D.C. His corporate career began with AMAF Industries in Washington D.C. conducting fundamental studies regarding the conversion of solar energy into electrical energy and the development of photoelectrochemical devices. While at Marconi GEC in Atlanta, GA he worked on catalyst designed to extend the lifetime of carbon dioxide TEA lasers. His efforts at Digital Equipment Corporation (DEC) In Andover, MA involved the development of advanced concepts for printed circuit boards and micro substrates. His responsibilities also included advanced material design and characterization; theoretical design of engineered polymers; and the development of advanced techniques utilizing laser beams and particle beams for fabrication of micro substrates.

The downsizing of America has found Dr. Conley becoming an independent consultant branching out into other fields. Over the last twenty years he has developed considerable expertise as a nutritional consultant. He designs diets, conducts workshops and lectures. He has concluded that the single greatest contributory factor in the high level of sickness and disease in America is over "consumption" or simply eating to much. The second greatest factor is excessive levels of meat in the diet followed by over eating of processed and refined grains. Dr. Conley recommends supplementation of certain nutrients, even when a good diet is followed. He has identified vitamin C and vitamin D as the two vitamins most important to human health. Vitamin C because of its central role in body defenses and the large amount required for optimal wellness. Vitamin D because it is needed for bone health and every cell and is supplied by very few foods.